MICHAEL GETS THE MEASLES

NOTEWORTHY BOOKS

MUSICAL BOOKS FOR YOUNG PEOPLE

THE ALPHABET OF MUSIC
THE BEAT OF THE DRUM
FOLK INSTRUMENTS
FOLLOW THE LEADER *[Story of Conducting]*
THE HEART OF THE ORCHESTRA *[Story of Strings]*
KEYBOARD INSTRUMENTS
PLACES OF MUSICAL FAME
PLAYBACK: THE STORY OF RECORDING DEVICES
SHINING BRASS *[Story of Trumpet and Brass]*
THE STORY OF MUSICAL NOTES
THE STORY OF MUSICAL ORGANIZATIONS
THE WOODWINDS

MEDICAL BOOKS FOR CHILDREN AND YOUNG PEOPLE

DEAR LITTLE MUMPS CHILD
DENTISTS' TOOLS
DOCTORS' TOOLS
FUR, FEATHERS, HAIR
HOW WE HEAR *[Story of Hearing]*
KAREN GETS A FEVER
LEFTY *[Story of Left-Handedness]*
MICHAEL GETS THE MEASLES
PENNY THE MEDICINE MAKER *[Story of Penicillin]*
PETER GETS THE CHICKENPOX
RED MAN, WHITE MAN, AFRICAN CHIEF
[Story of Skin Color]
THEY WOULDN'T QUIT *[Story of Handicapped]*
TWINS *[Story of Twins]*
WHY GLASSES? *[Story of Vision]*

MR. BUMBA BOOKS
[Easy Reading]

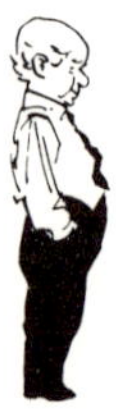

MR. BUMBA'S NEW HOME
MR. BUMBA PLANTS A GARDEN
MR. BUMBA KEEPS HOUSE
MR. BUMBA AND THE ORANGE GROVE
MR. BUMBA'S NEW JOB
MR. BUMBA HAS A PARTY

The above books are written by competent authorities and attractively illustrated. Information about obtaining these is available from

Lerner Publications Company
133 FIRST AVENUE NORTH
MINNEAPOLIS 1, MINNESOTA

Michael Gets the Measles

By Marguerite Rush Lerner, M. D.

Illustrated by George Overlie

MEDICAL BOOKS FOR CHILDREN
Minneapolis 1, Minnesota

Fourth Printing 1963, Fifth Printing 1964

Library of Congress Catalog Number: 59-13630. Third Printing 1961.

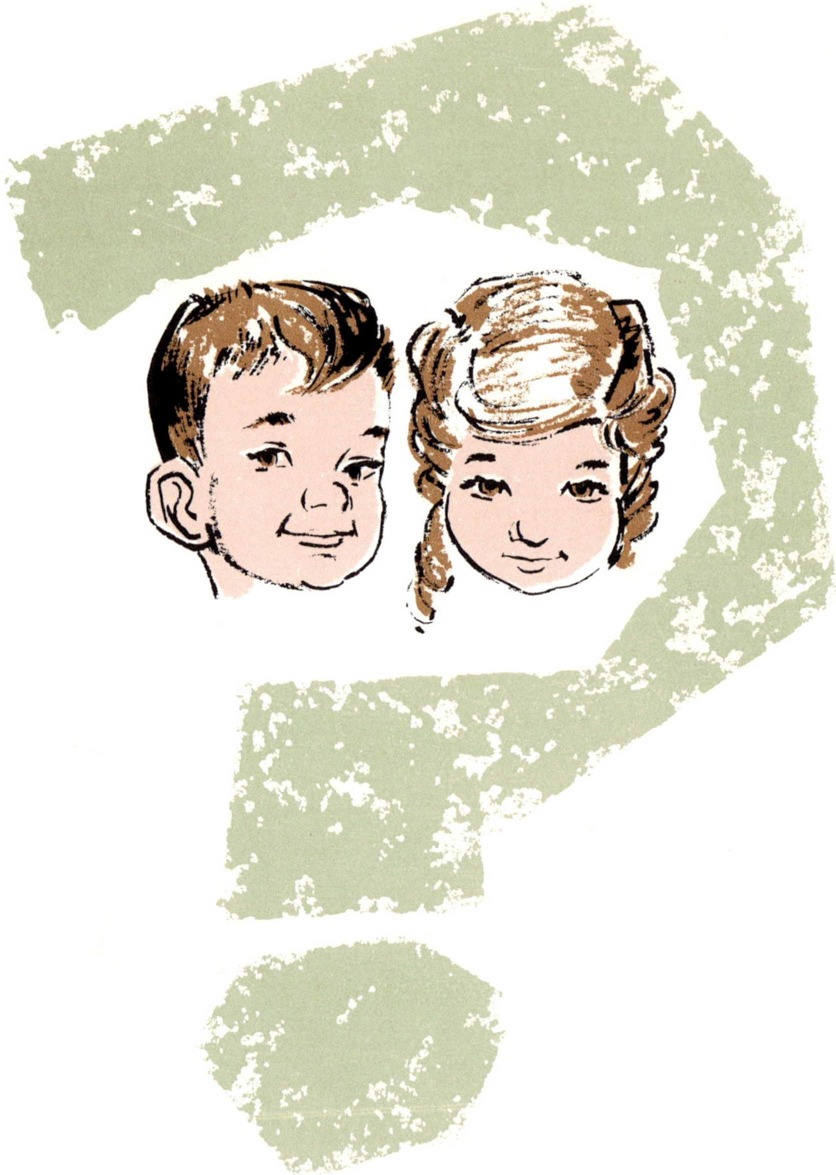

Did you ever have the measles?

Did your nose get sniffly sneezy?
Did your eyes turn pinkish red?
And every time you tried to talk,
did a cough come out instead?

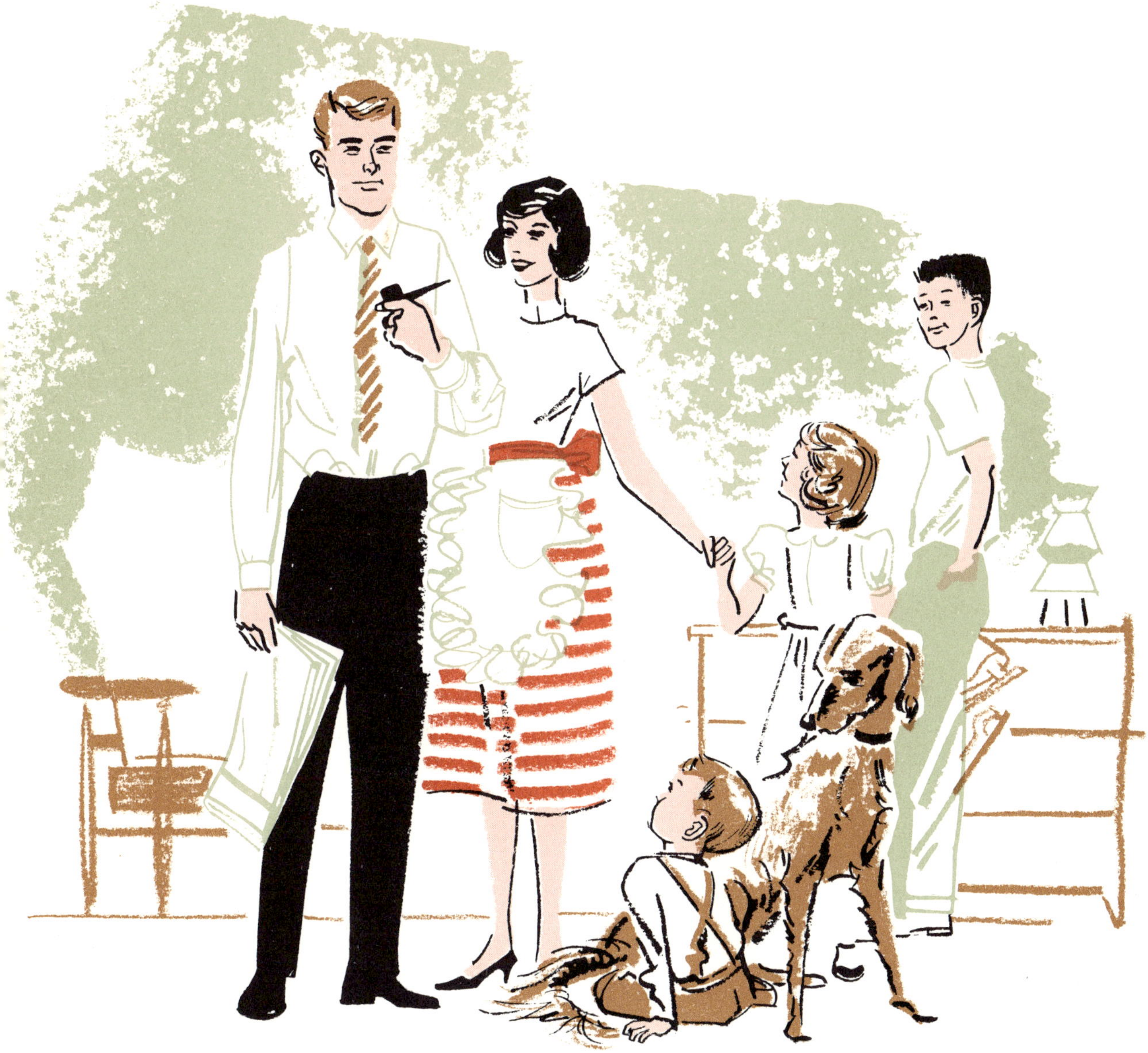

That is just what happened to Michael.

Michael was a boy four years old.
He had a sister and a brother,
a father and a mother,
and a dog named Rusty.

Michael liked to go to nursery school
where a boy named Hugh was his special friend.
As soon as Mike saw Hugh he'd say,
"Hi, Hugh! So it's *you* again!"

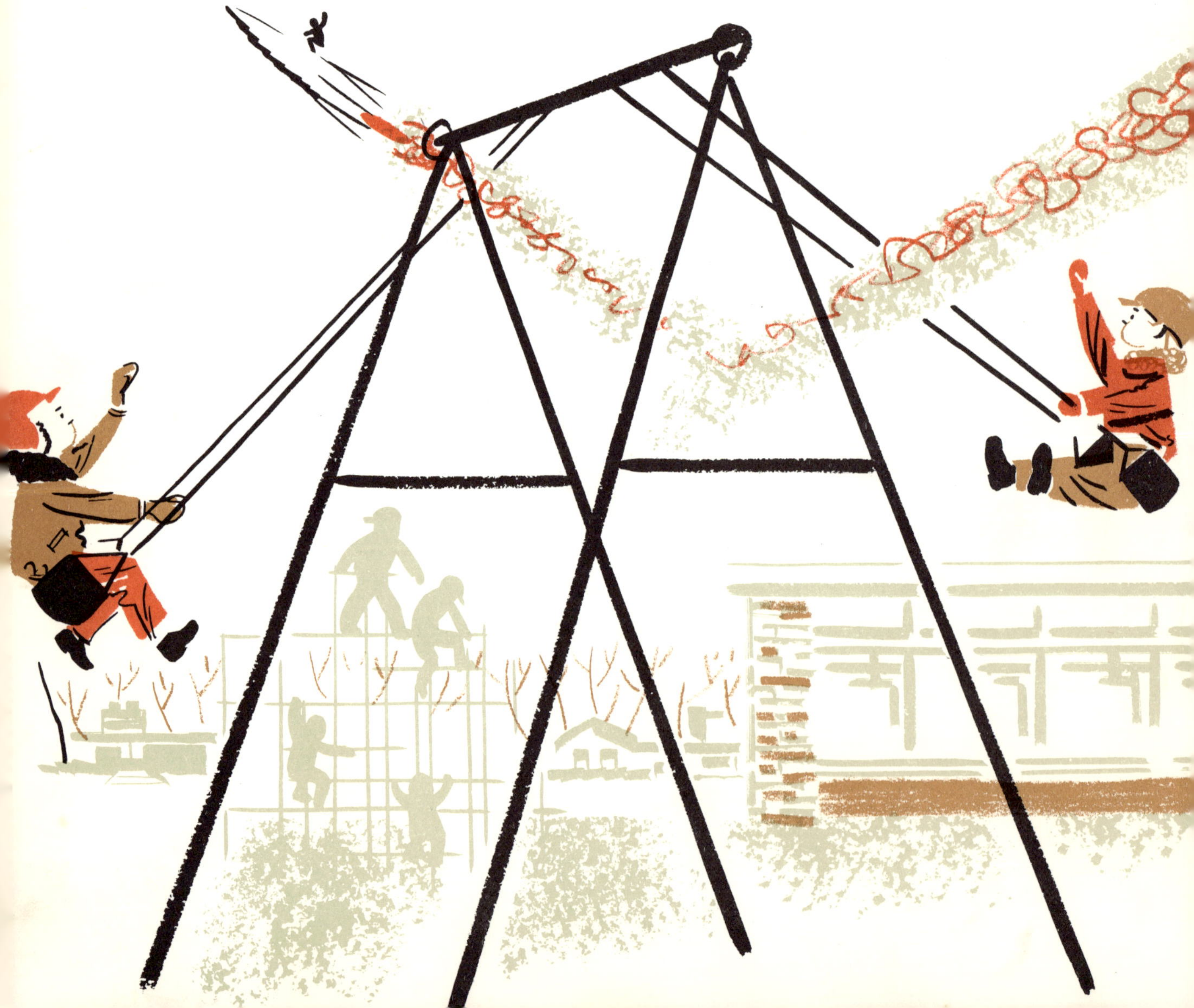

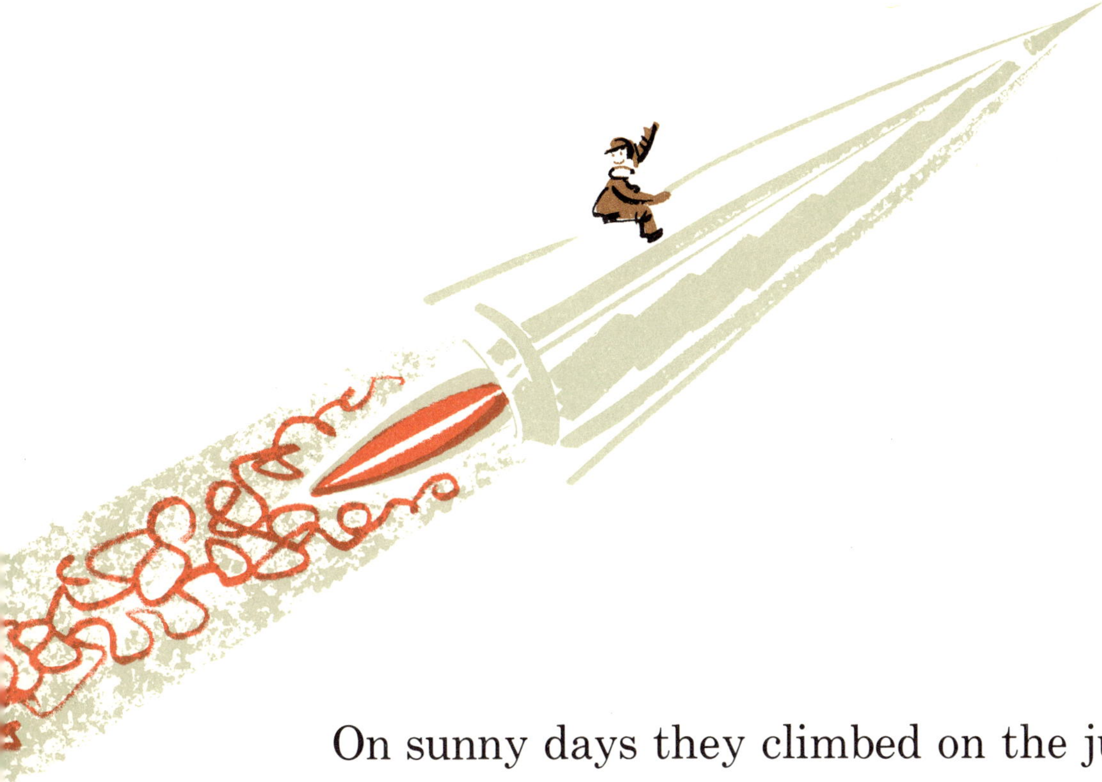

On sunny days they climbed on the jungle gym,
swung on the swings,
pretended they were pilots
on rockets without wings.

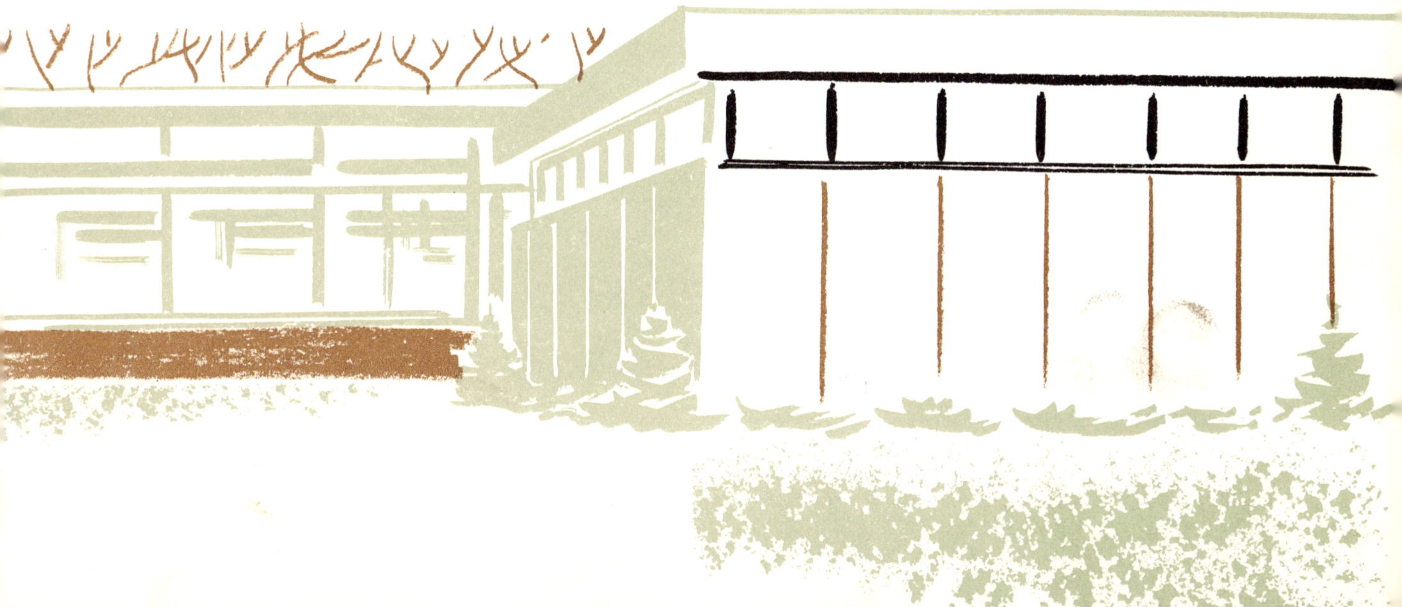

On rainy days there were other things to do.
They painted at a painting easel – Michael and Hugh.
With splashes of red and yellow and green
they covered the paper till no white could be seen.

One day when Michael went to school
he couldn't find his friend named Hugh.
He wasn't outside anywhere.
Michael looked inside – was he there?

No.
Where was he?
Michael's teacher said,
"Hugh has the measles
and is home in bed."

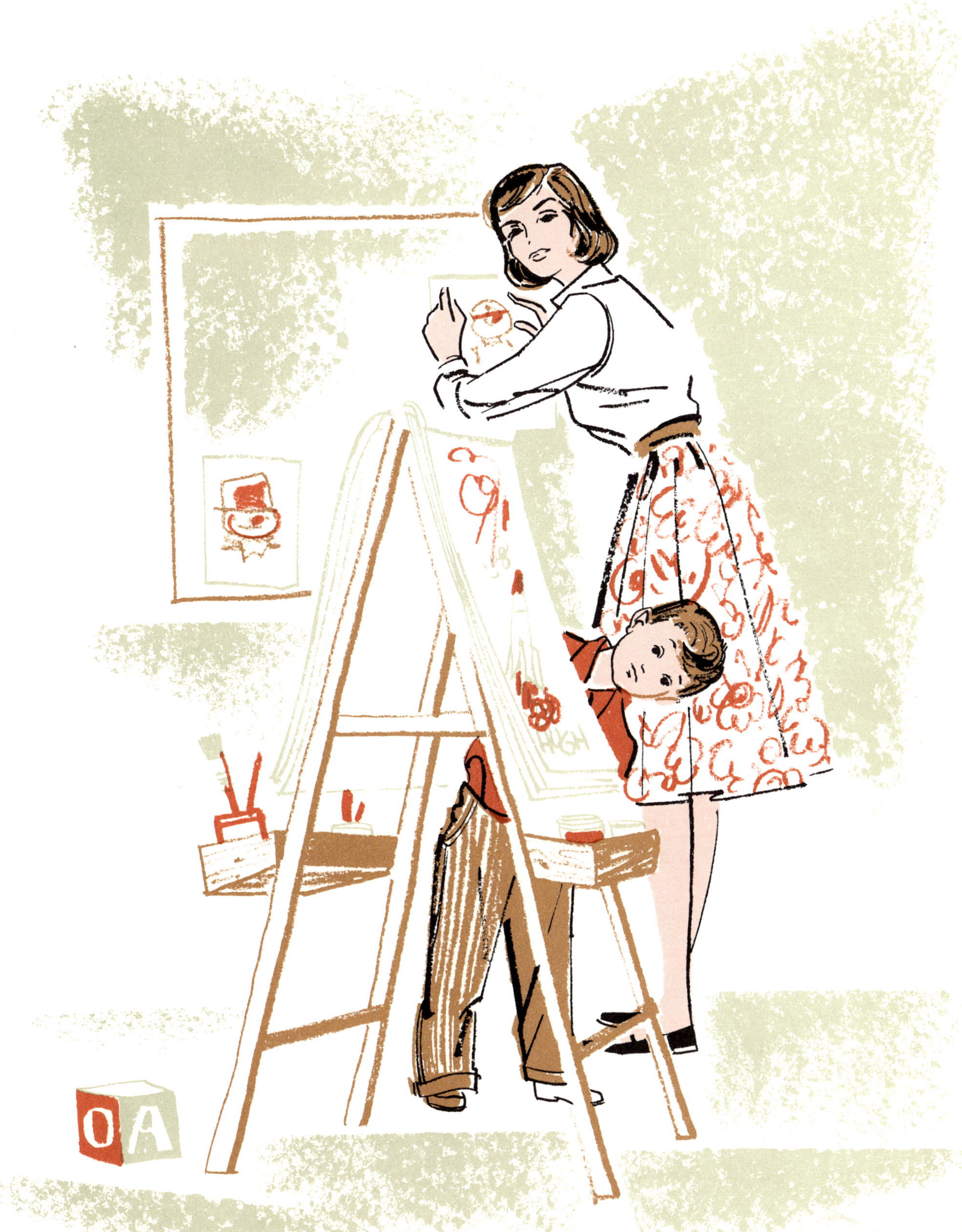

About ten mornings after that
Michael woke up and cried,
"I don't feel so pretty good.
I think I'm sick inside."

Michael's mother took a thermometer,
which is a special kind of stick
used to measure temperature
when you are feeling sick.

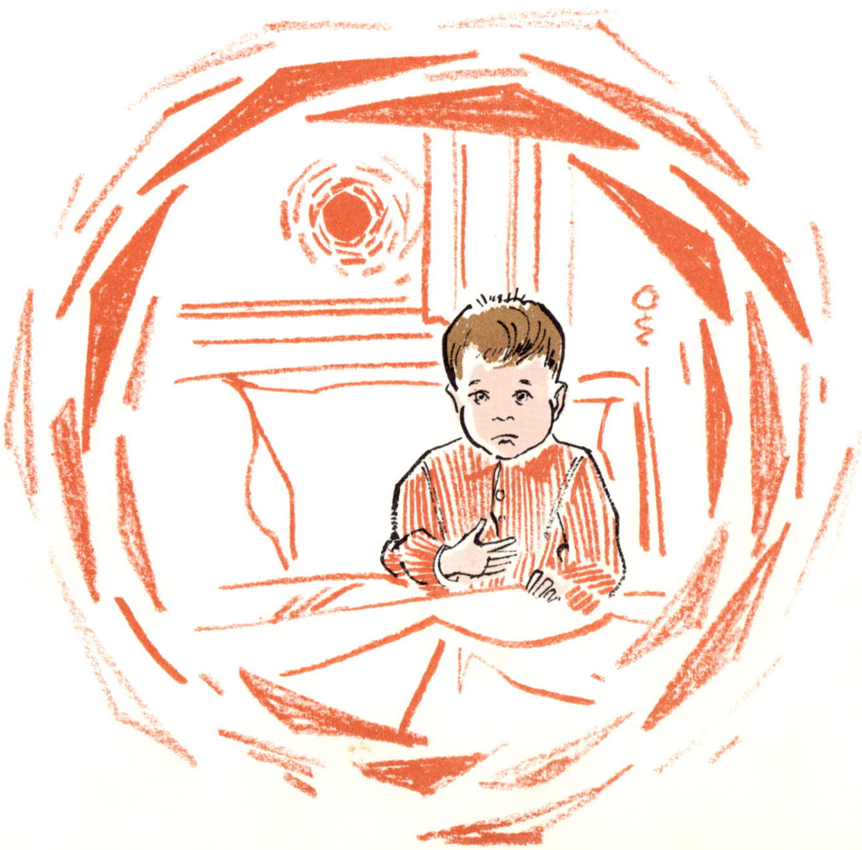

She said, "Lie down for three minutes."
"Three minutes – how long is that?"
Michael asked his mother
while up in bed he sat.

"Lie still," she said
"and count to ten
18 times
and that's the end."

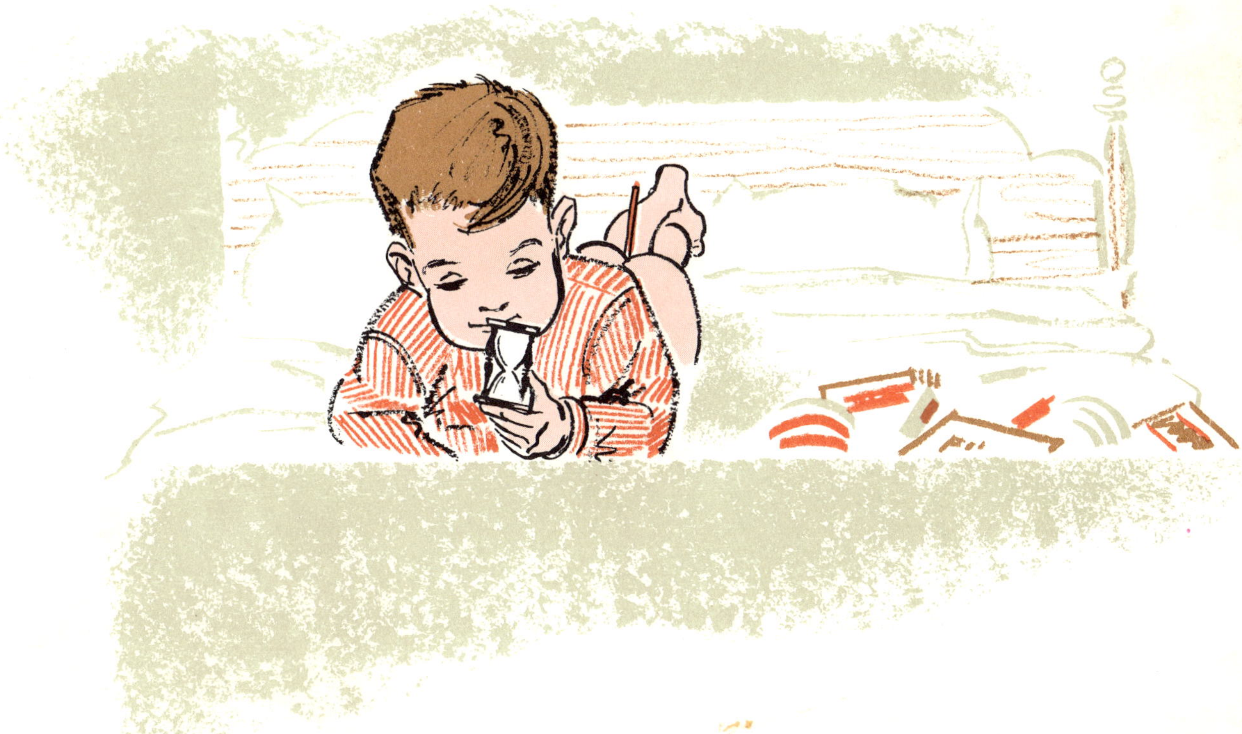

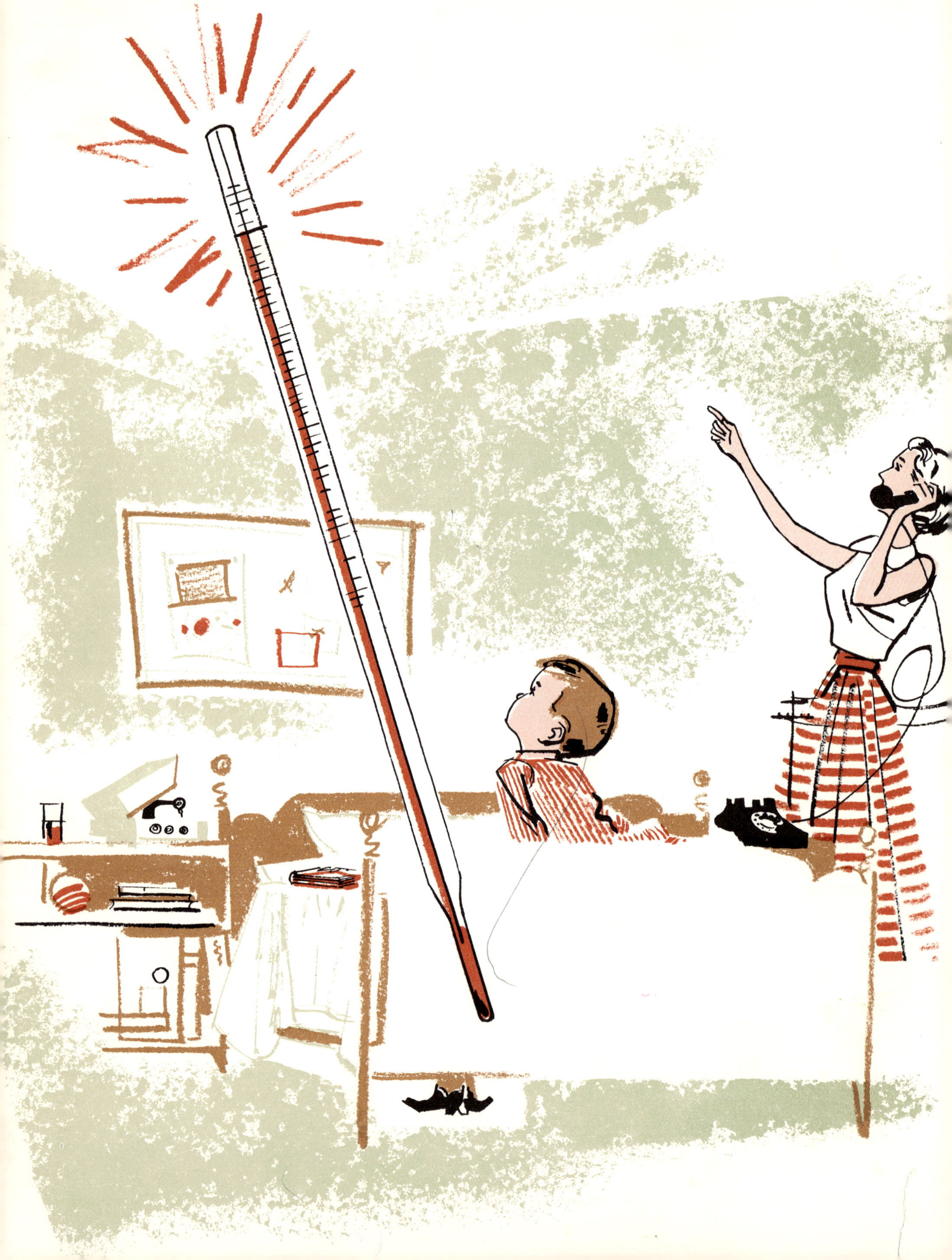

The thermometer read 101 degrees,

which means a fever, though not too much.

However, it's enough to stay home from school,

work puzzles, listen to records, read books and such.

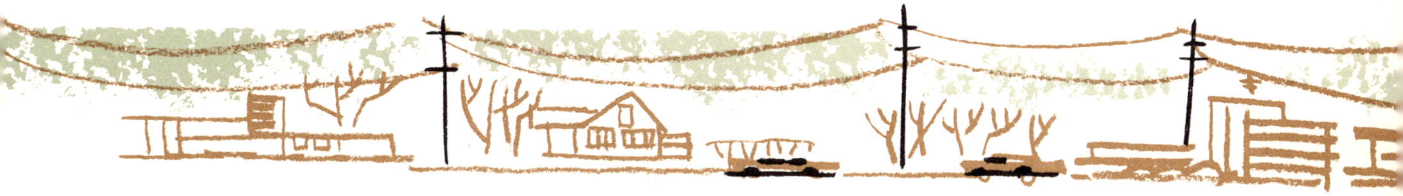

The next day Michael's temperature was normal.

He really didn't seem sick.

BUT THE DAY AFTER THAT

the thermometer shot way past 98 point six.

His nose was sniffly sneezy,
his eyes were pinkish red,
and every time he tried to talk
a cough came out instead.

Michael's mother snuggled him in a blanket,
then called Dr. Paul on the phone.
"Michael is sick with a cough and cold and fever.
Can you come see him at our home?"

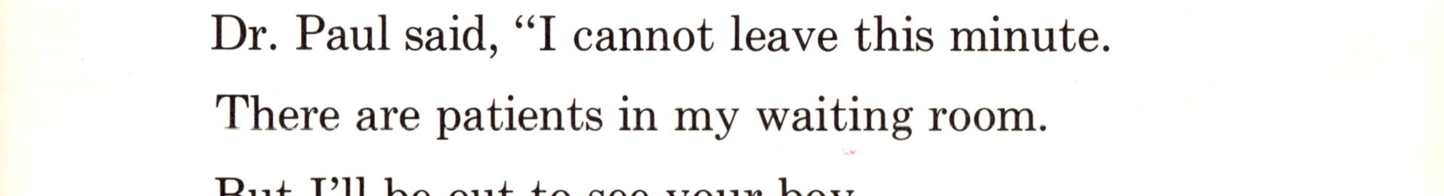

Dr. Paul said, "I cannot leave this minute.
There are patients in my waiting room.
But I'll be out to see your boy
sometime this afternoon.

"Give him an aspirin for his fever.
Keep him comfortable in bed.
Measles are going around just now
so watch for skin spots that are red."

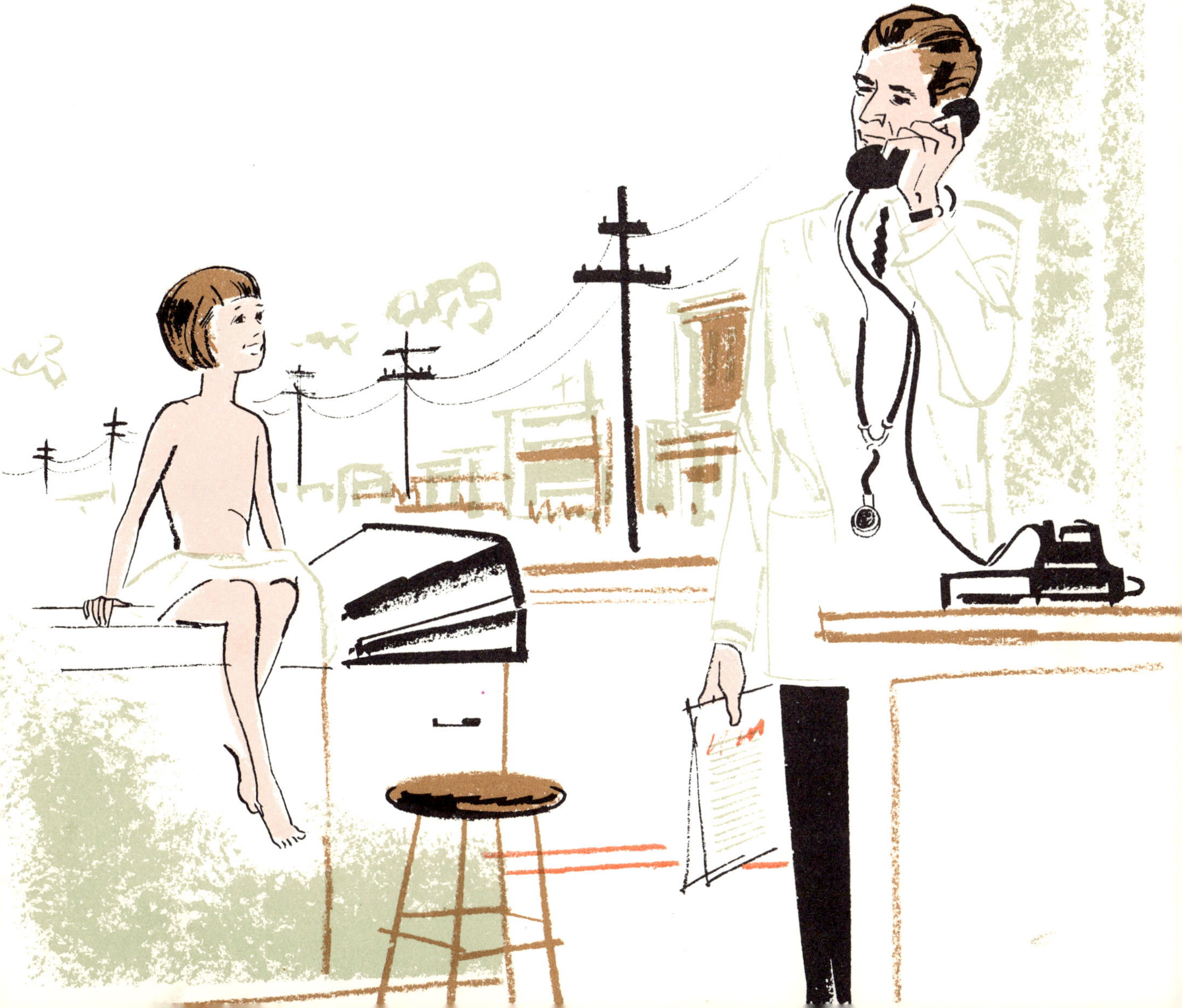

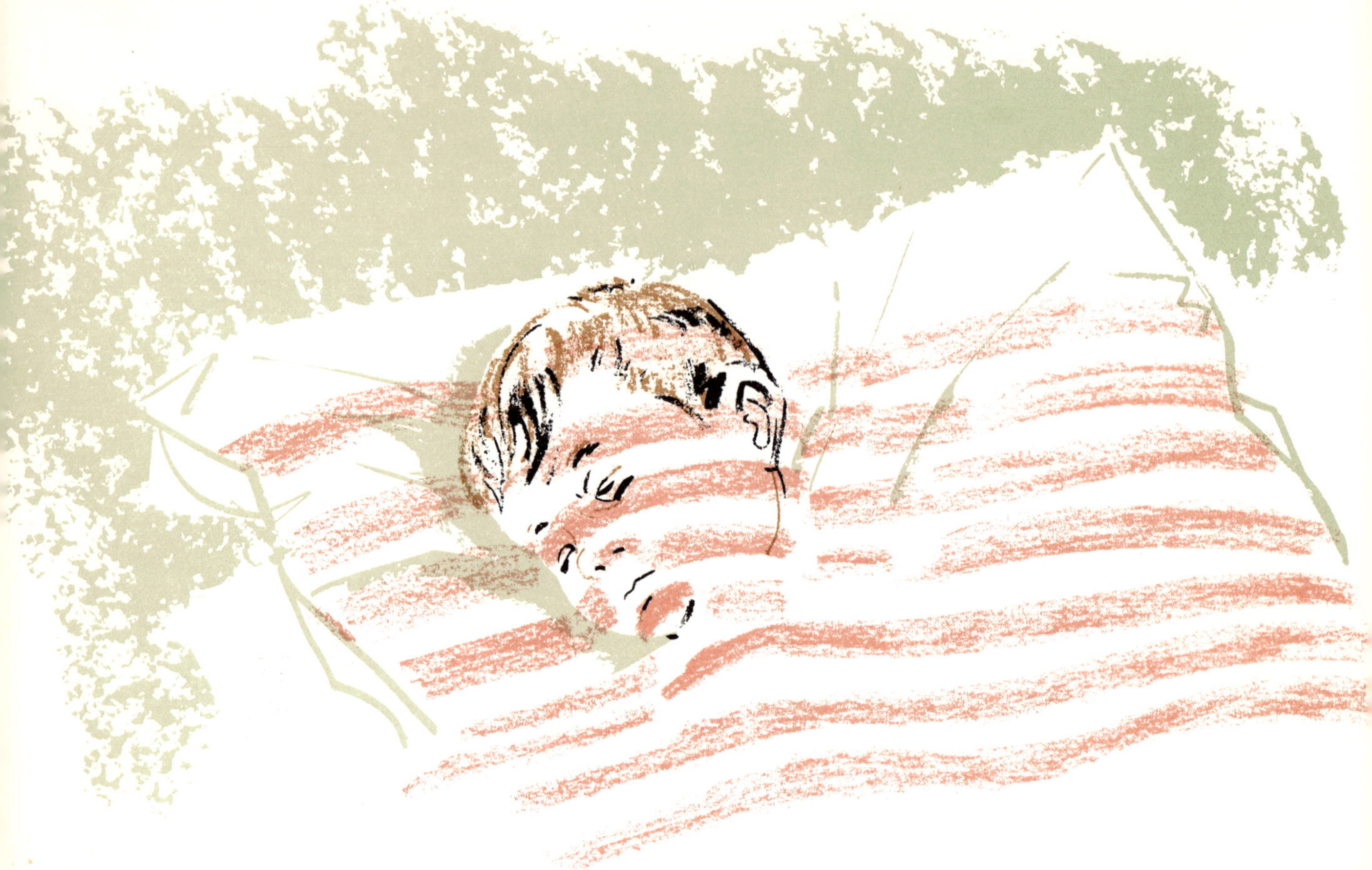

As the morning hours dragged on,

Michael felt sick and even sicker.

The sun that shone from outside in

seemed to make his eyelids flicker.

At last the door bell rang.

The doctor came.

He looked in Michael's eyes

with a shiny silvery light.

"I don't think I like that," Michael said,

"Your light is much too bright."

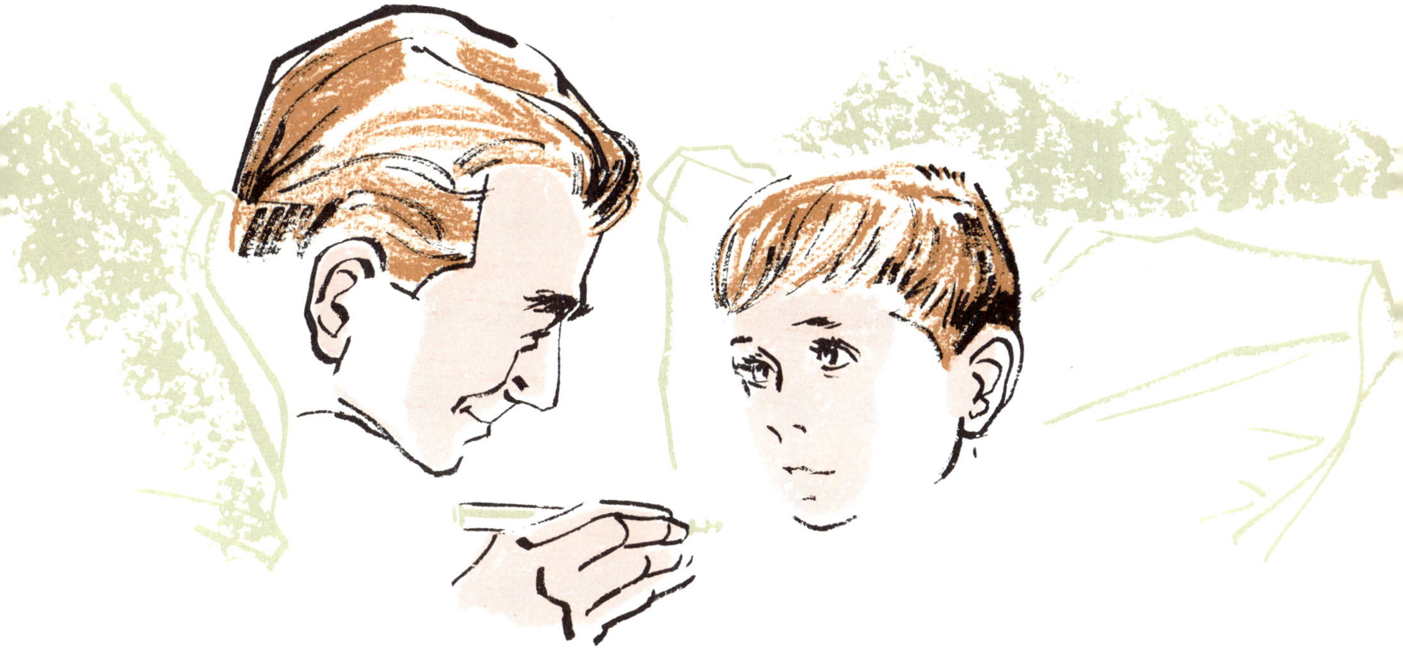

Then Michael sneezed and wheezed and coughed.

Dr. Paul said, "You just sit and rest

while I take my stethoscope

and listen to your chest.

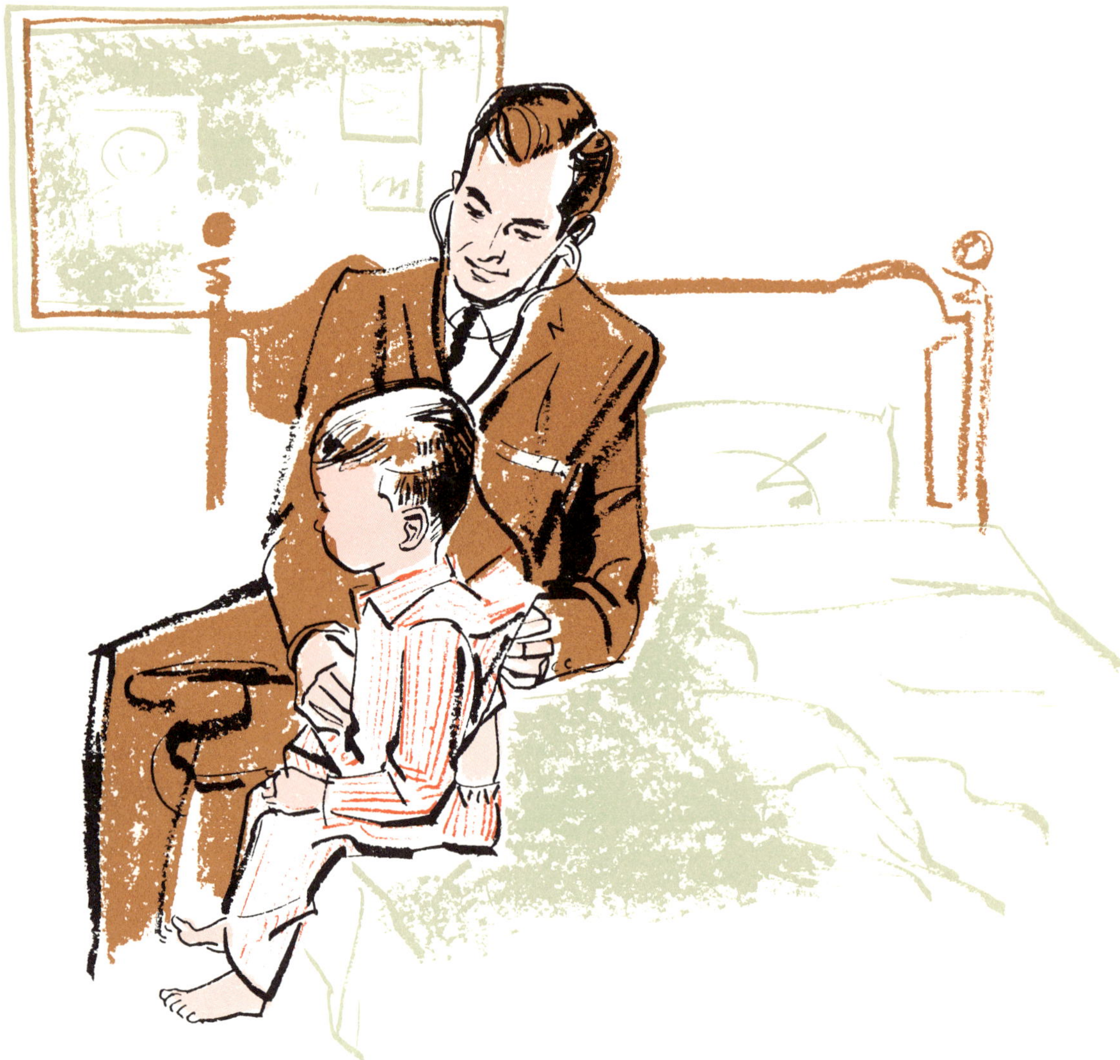

"Can you pretend that you're a dog?
Open up your mouth.
Now pant like a puppy that's run a race
so the air goes in and out."

Michael breathed as he was told
so the air went in and out.
Dr. Paul said, "Your chest is fine.
"Now let's look inside your mouth.

"Hmm," the doctor said,
inspecting Michael's mouth.
"Michael's got the measles.
Of that there is no doubt."

"How can that be?" asked Michael's mother.
"Measles without red spots?
Shouldn't there be a few at least,
and maybe even lots?"

"Maybe it's the geasles,"
Michael interjected.
"Or maybe it's the chickenpox
that's got me all infected."

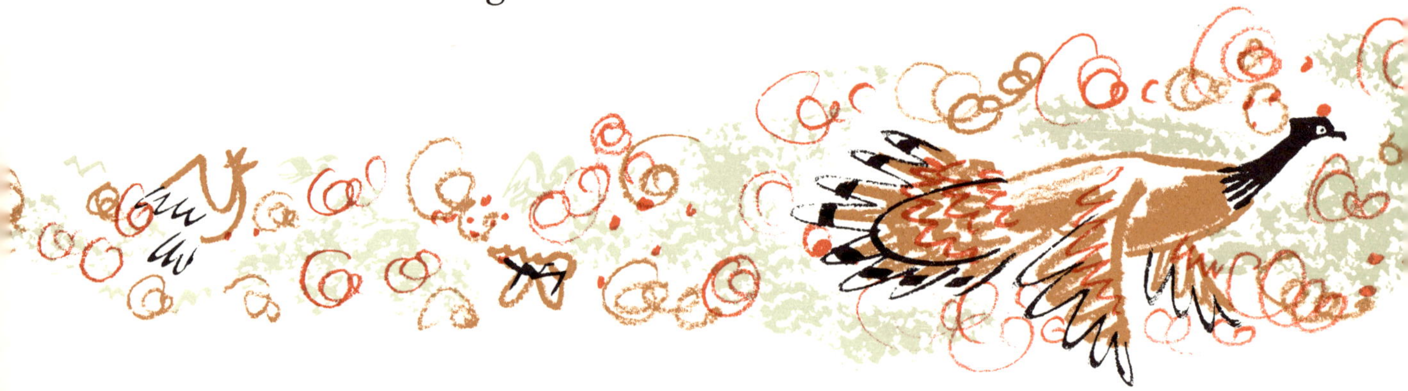

"It can't be geasles
because there's no such thing.
And it can't be the chickenpox –
you had them last spring!"

Then Michael said,
"Maybe I've got
the turkeypox!"
But whoever heard of the turkeypox?

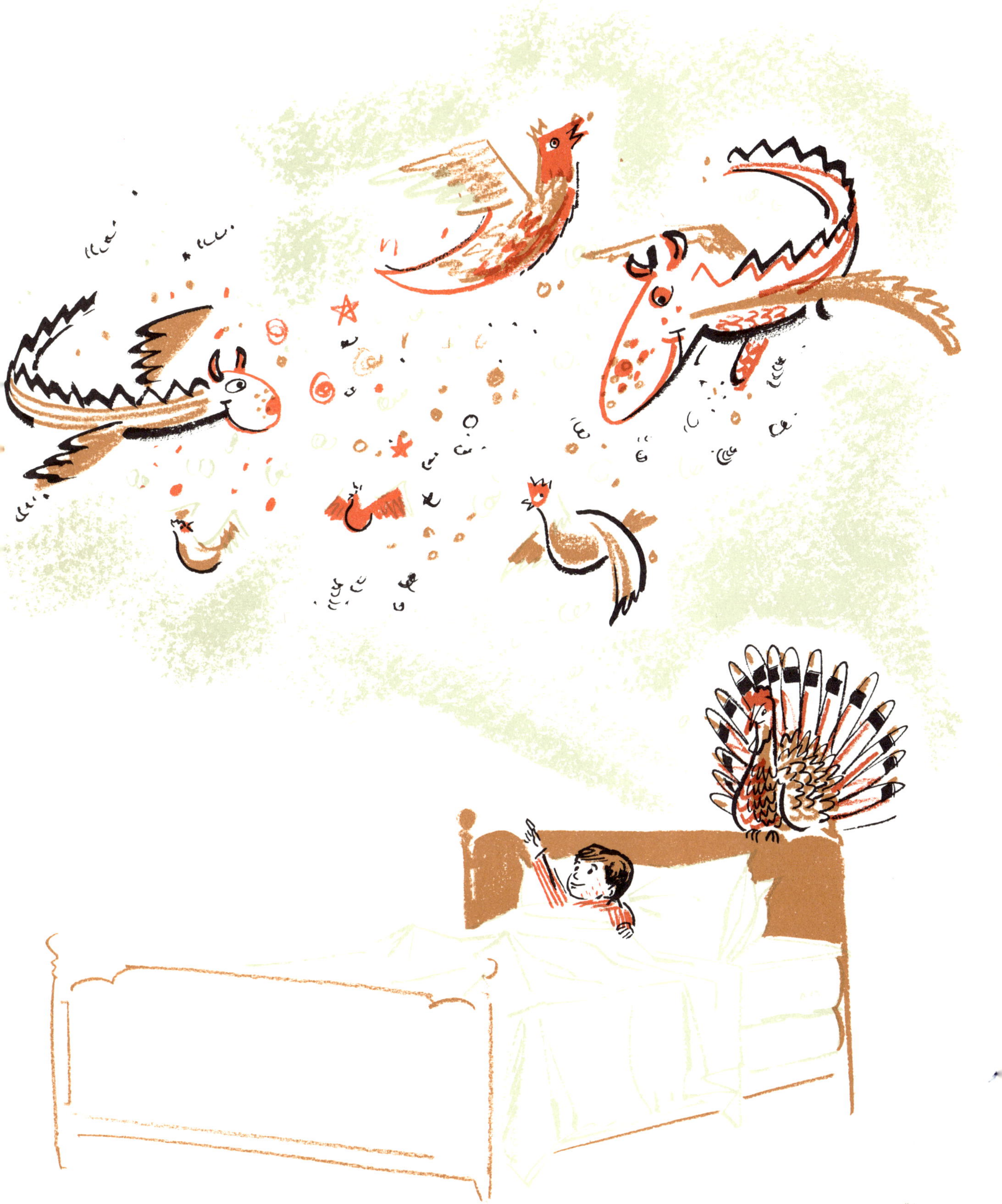

"Let me tell you why it's measles,"

the doctor politely said.

"Inside of Michael's cheeks and lips

are specks of white and red.

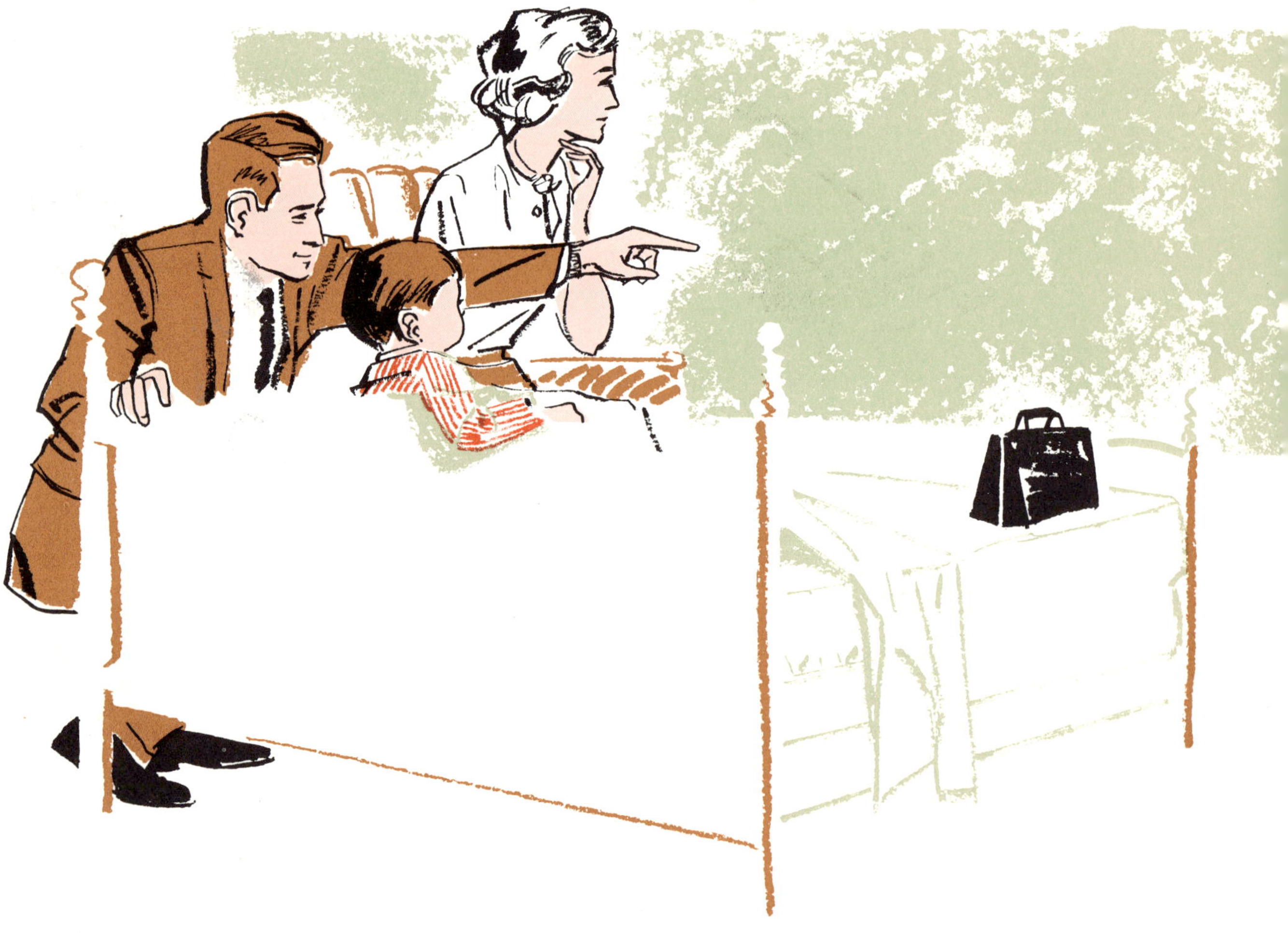

"When these specks,
called Koplik's spots, appear,
we know that the measles rash
is very near.

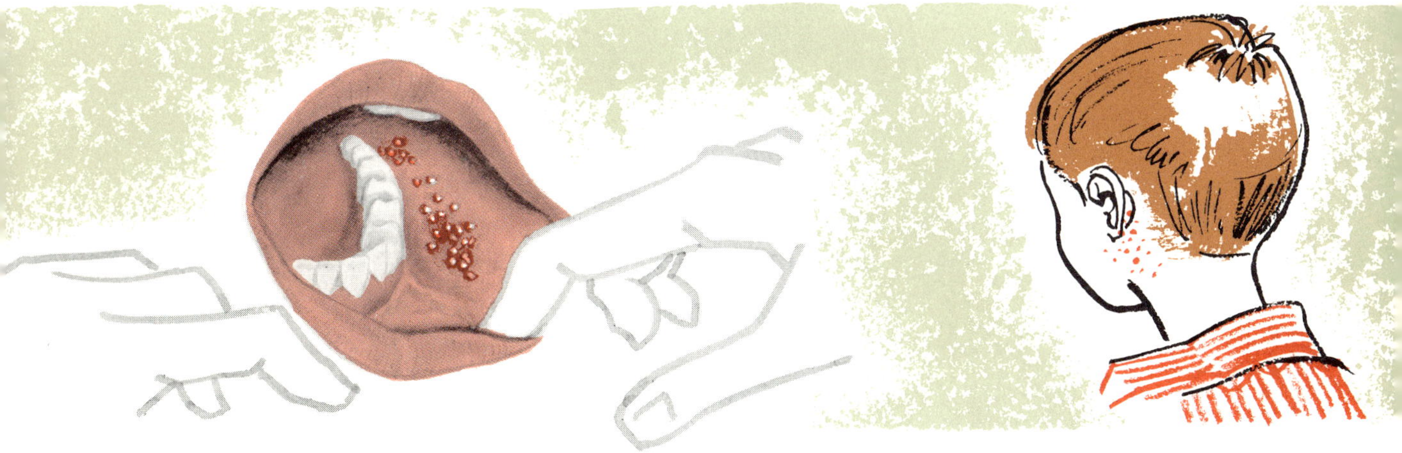

"Call me in the morning.
Let me know if Mike's all right."
Then guess what happened? Behind Mike's ears
spots came out that very night.

By morning time Michael's mother
knew the doctor was correct,
for red spots had appeared
along the sides of Michael's neck.

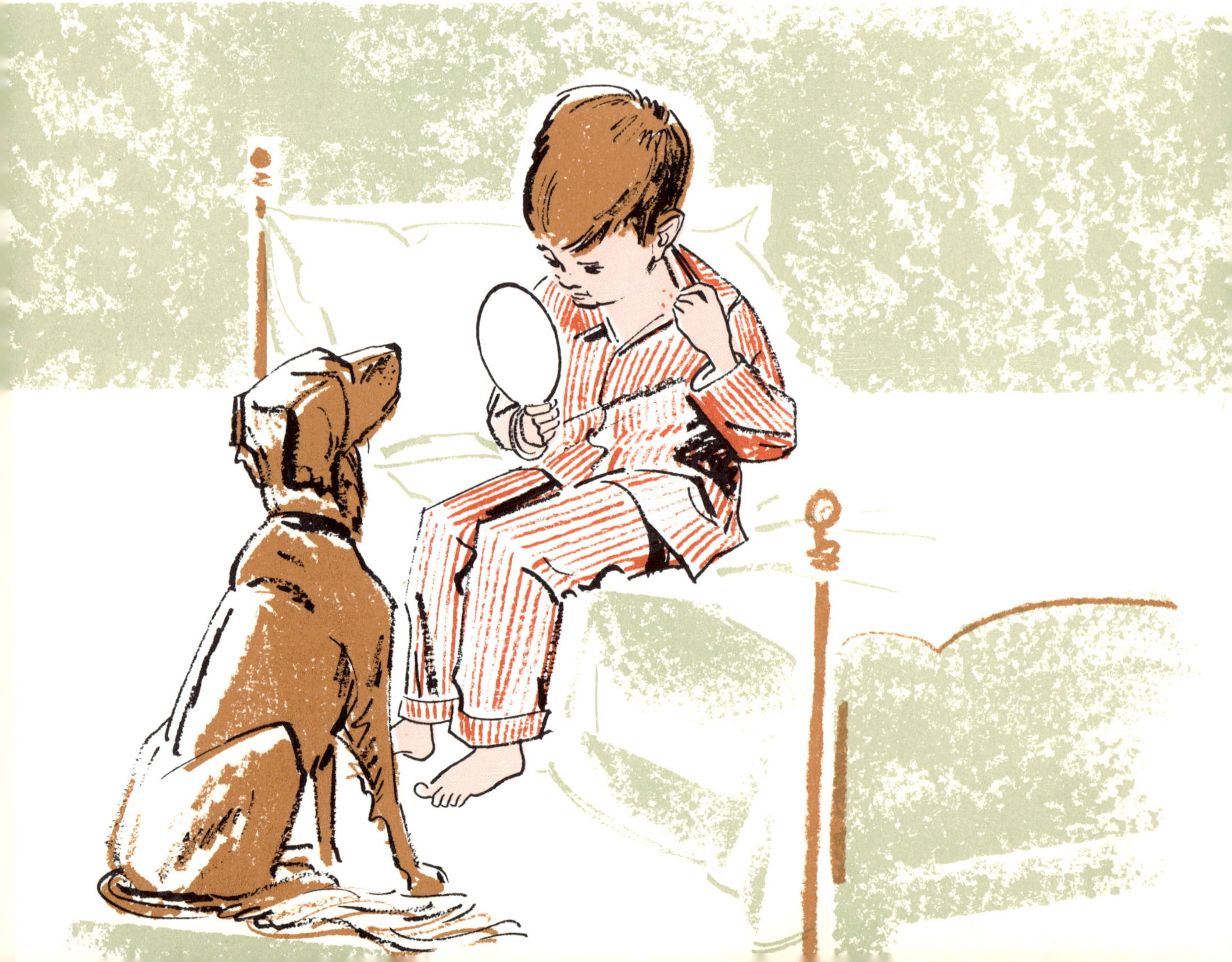

The cheeks and face
began to sprout
the tiny measly spots of red —
before the afternoon was out.

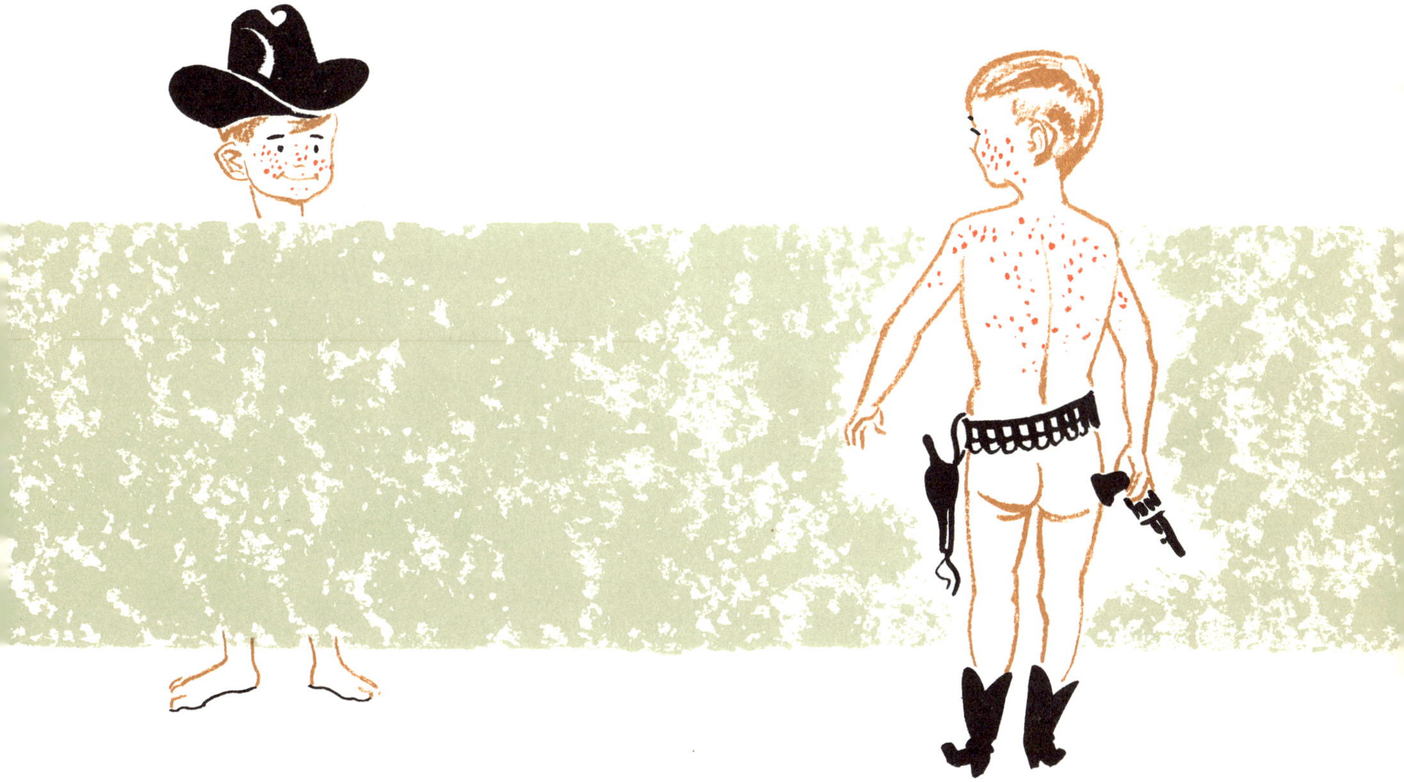

By night time the upper arms and chest
also were getting spotted.
And the morning after,
Michael's back became quite dotted.

By afternoon the lower part of
Michael's arms looked funny.
And by that night
there were spots across his tummy.

Meanwhile, as the rash appeared,
Michael felt worse, not better.
His fever rose, he coughed and coughed,
and his eyes got even redder.

The third day after it had started,
the rash began to spread
down down Michael's body,
down down to his legs,
until it reached
both his feet.

Then something happened.

His fever stopped.
His cough got small.
His eyes didn't look
red at all.

The skin rash changed in color

from red to copper like a penny.

Then it turned brown.

Then there wasn't any!

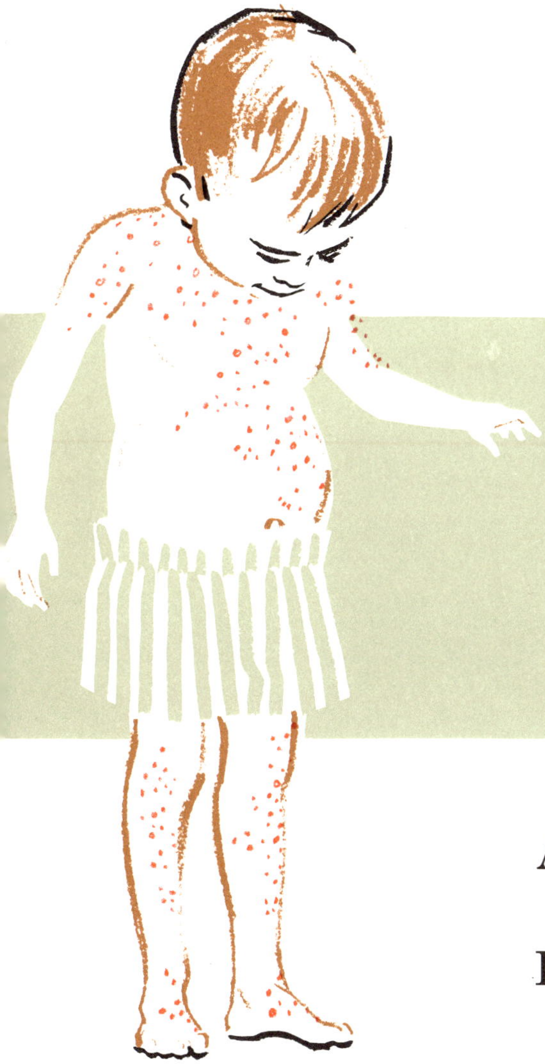

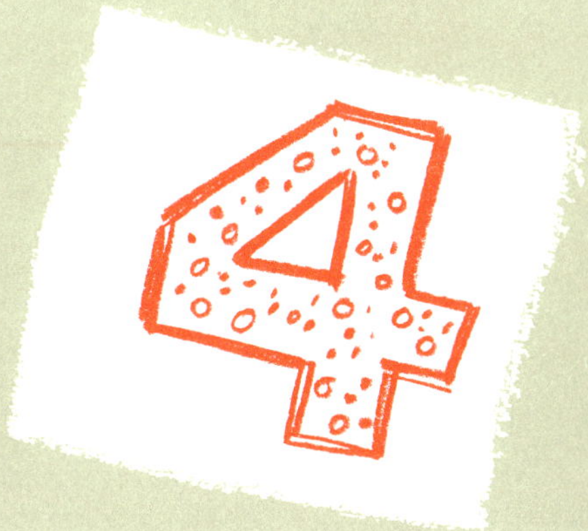

A measles rash is not so bad.

It isn't half as itchy

as the blister bumps of chickenpox

which feel so scratchy-scritchy.

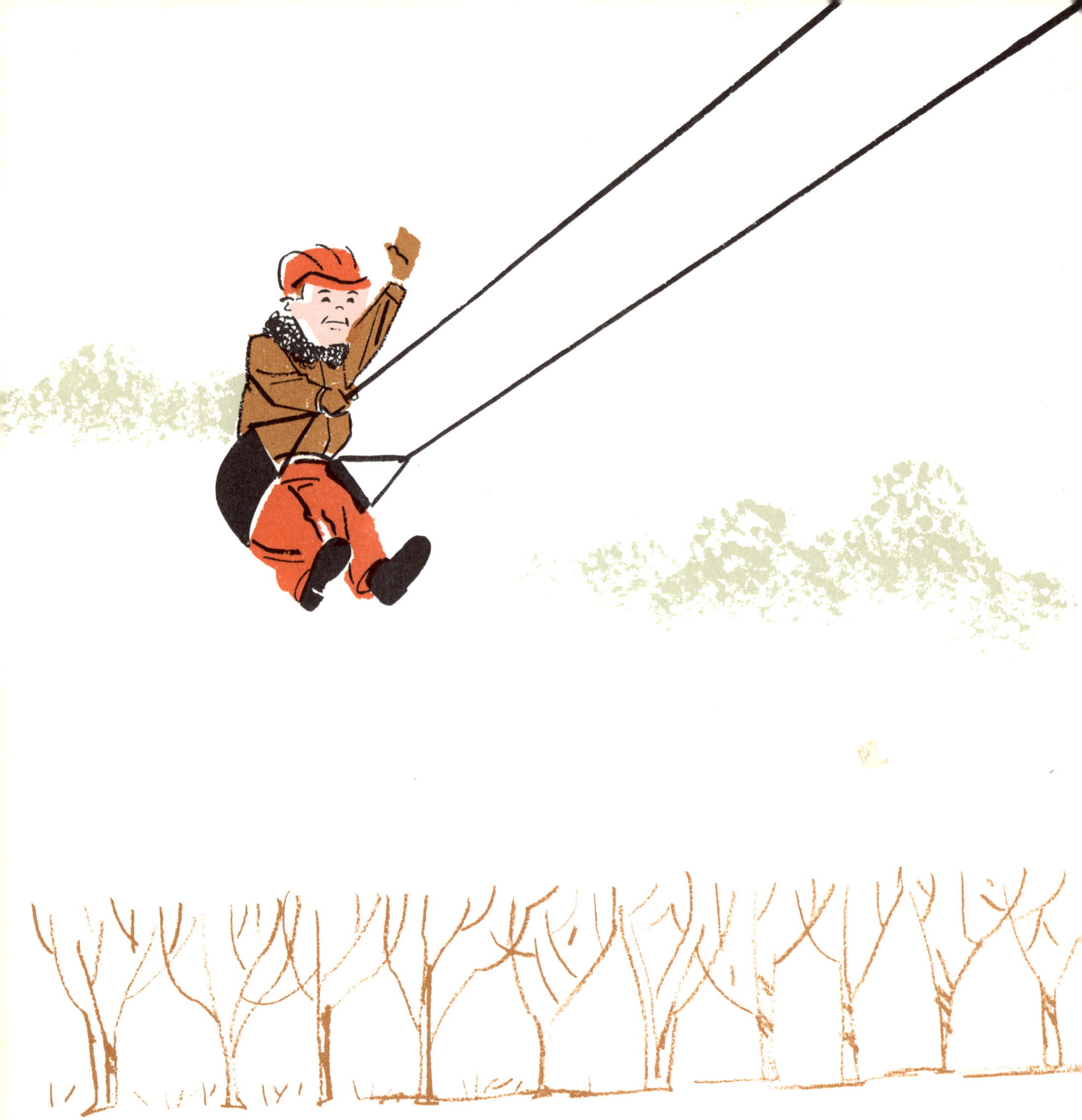

Michael was well and back at school
one week after the measles began.
He looked outside and inside
till he found Hugh, his friend.

Hugh looked at Mike and cried,
"Hi, Mike! so it's *you* again!"
And Michael answered Hugh,
"Guess what? I had the measles, too."

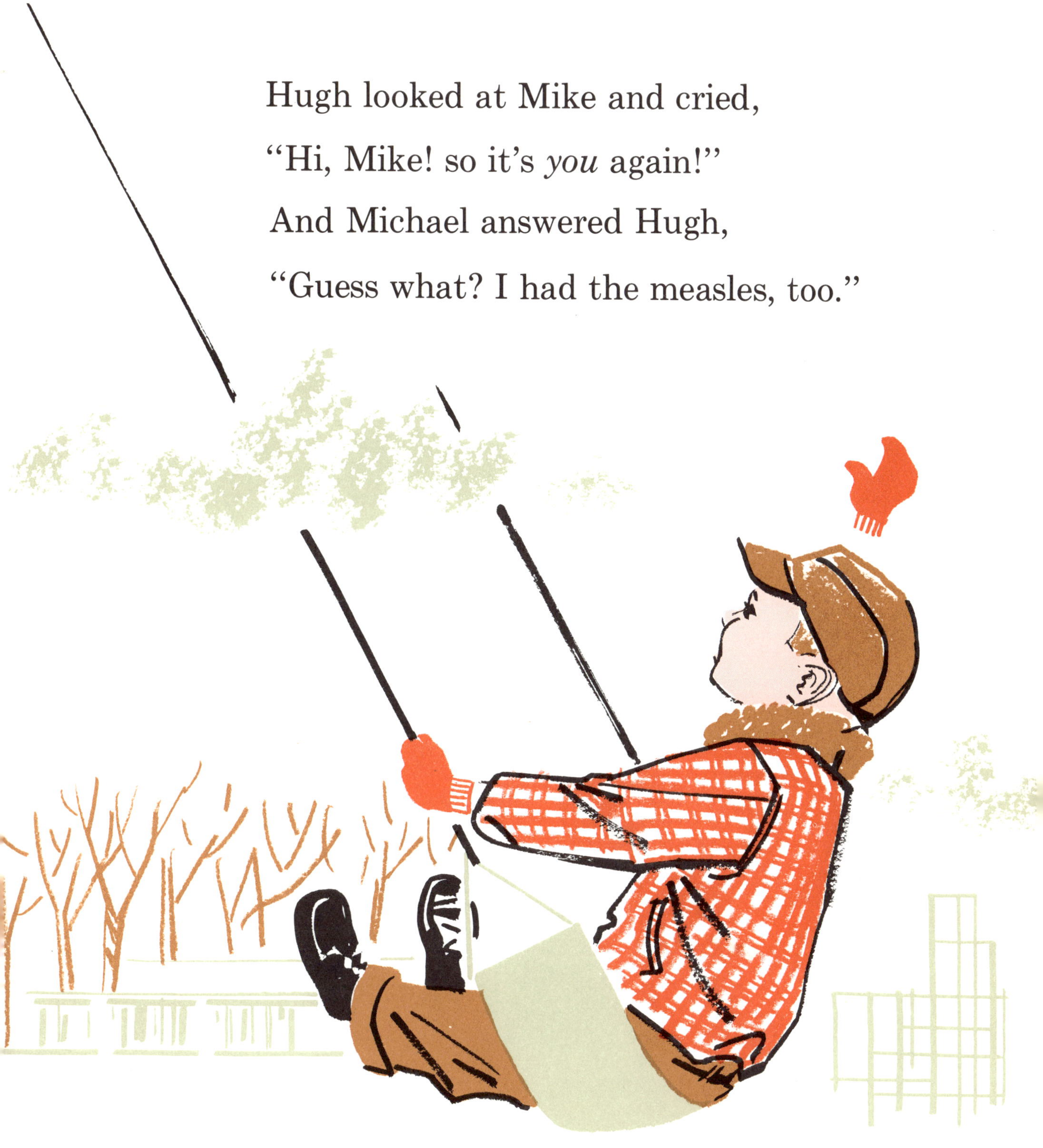

You can walk 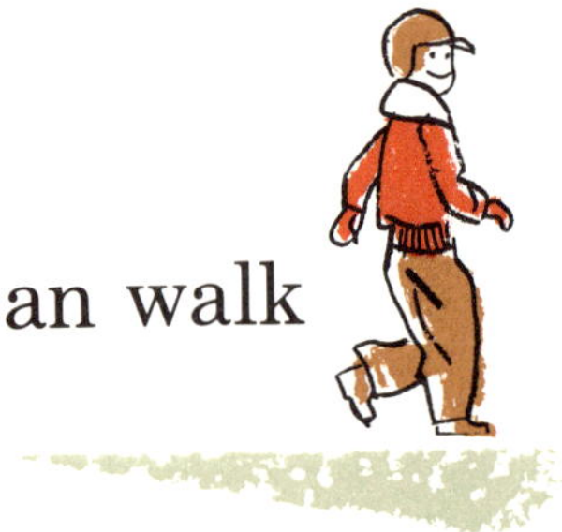 and you can run. 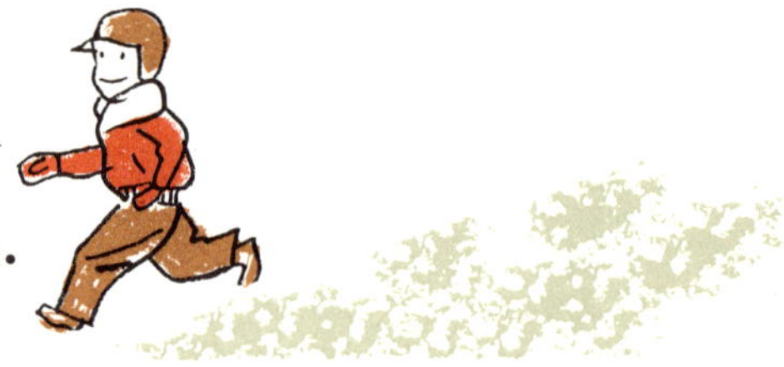

But once the measles have begun,

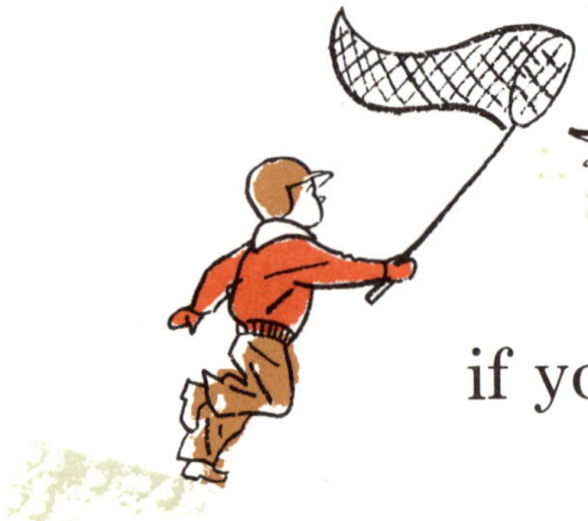

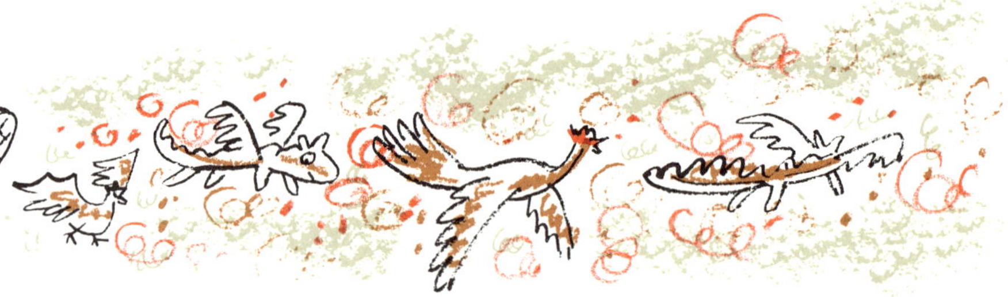

if you don't catch the measles

the measles will catch you!"

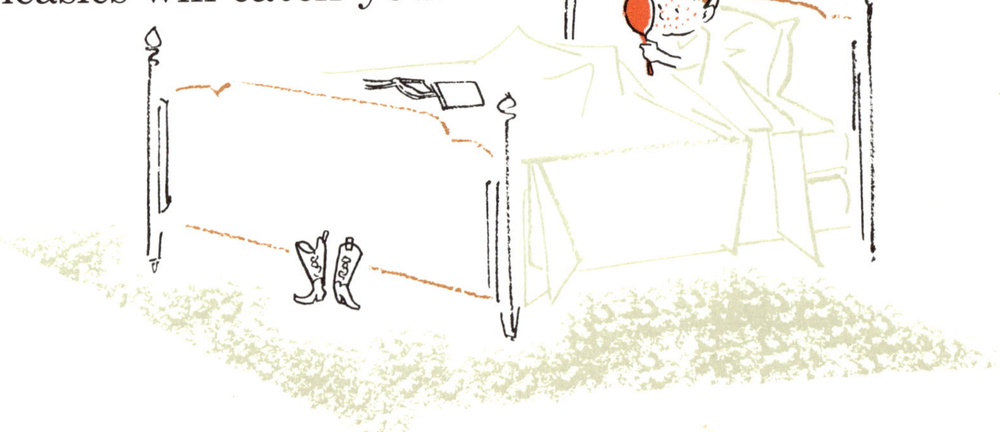

INFORMATION FOR PARENTS AND TEACHERS

THE NAME The word measles is derived from the Middle English *mesels*, a variation of *maseles*, and means little spot or speck. An old Latin name for measles was *morbilli*, for little illness. The medical name for ordinary measles is rubeola, which comes from the Latin *ruber* for ruby or red. German measles is called rubella.

ETIOLOGY Measles is an infectious disease caused by a virus. Under the electron microscope the measles virus appears roughly circular with a diameter of 1,200 to 2,500 angstroms – about 1/30th the diameter of a red blood cell. The virus is of the RNA type and is similar in structure to other large members of the myxovirus group such as mumps.

AGE INCIDENCE Measles is chiefly a disease of childhood.

SEX AND RACE Both sexes and all races are equally susceptible.

SEASONS Before the measles vaccine became available, measles occurred in epidemics at two- to four-year intervals and also in between.

CONTAGIOUSNESS Measles is highly contagious and is spread through the air as well as by direct contact with infectious material produced by sneezing, coughing or talking. The virus is particularly communicable during the early stage of sneezing, coughing and runny nose. Measles is less contagious after the rash develops. Before the vaccine was used, 90% of children under the age of six who had not had measles got it during the first epidemic to which they were exposed. The rest developed measles during a subsequent epidemic. Hence, most people caught measles before reaching adulthood.

(continued)

INCUBATION PERIOD The time required after exposure to a patient with measles until the rash appears in a susceptible person is from 12 to 19 days. However, the incubation period between exposure and development of first symptoms—such as fever, sneezing, runny nose, red eyes, cough — is 10 days. These early symptoms come one to five days before the rash. Koplik or mouth spots appear one to four days before onset of the rash.

COMPLICATIONS Measles lasts about one week. Complications are not common but can be severe. If after the rash has faded fever occurs, or there are complaints of earache, headache, nausea, vomiting, persistent cough or increasing cough, the doctor should be called.

TREATMENT There is no treatment for the measles virus itself. Once measles has occurred, aspirin can be given for fever, and a cough syrup may be recommended by the physician. The severity of the disease in a susceptible person can be decreased by injection of gamma globulin within five days after exposure to a patient ill with measles. However, it is better to prevent measles by vaccination than to get the disease.

VACCINATION Measles vaccine was released for clinical trial in 1962, and soon after large scale immunizations were begun. In 1967 a program for mass eradication of measles was started, and about 25 million children were given the vaccine. The inoculated subjects did not get measles, and by 1968 measles had decreased 80% in the general population. In some states where nearly all the children were vaccinated, for example, in Rhode Island, measles has practically disappeared. Reactions to the measles vaccine are minimal and minor. A few persons develop fever and a rash but do not feel sick. Children should be inoculated when one year old.

IMMUNITY Immunity is usually lifelong following an attack of measles. Infants are immune to measles from birth till about six months of age. Injection of live, attenuated measles virus vaccine confers immunity in almost 100% of susceptible people. The exact duration of immunity following inoculation of measles vaccine is not known yet but is long lasting.